Theory at a Glance

A Guide For Health Promotion Practice
(Second Edition)

U.S. DEPARTMENT OF HEALTH AND HUMAN SERVICES
National Institutes of Health

Foreword

A decade ago, the first edition of *Theory at a Glance* was published. The guide was a welcome resource for public health practitioners seeking a single, concise summary of health behavior theories that was neither overwhelming nor superficial. As a government publication in the public domain, it also provided cash-strapped health departments with access to a seminal integration of scholarly work that was useful to program staff, interns, and directors alike. Although they were not the primary target audience, members of the public health research community also utilized *Theory at a Glance*, both as a quick desk reference and as a primer for their students.

The National Cancer Institute is pleased to sponsor the publication of this guide, but its relevance is by no means limited to cancer prevention and control. The principles described herein can serve as frameworks for many domains of public health intervention, complementing focused evidence reviews such as Centers for Disease Control and Prevention's *Guide to Community Preventive Services*. This report also complements a number of other efforts by NCI and our federal partners to facilitate more rigorous testing and application of health behavior theories through training workshops and the development of new Web-based resources.

One reason theory is so useful is that it helps us articulate assumptions and hypotheses concerning our strategies and targets of intervention. Debates among policymakers concerning public health programs are often complicated by unspoken assumptions or confusion about which data are relevant. Theory can inform these debates by clarifying key constructs and their presumed relationships. Especially when the evidence base is small, advocates of one approach or another can be challenged to address the mechanisms by which a program is expected to have an impact. By specifying these alternative pathways to change, program evaluations can be designed to ensure that regardless of the outcome, improvements in knowledge, program design, and implementation will occur.

I am pleased to introduce this second edition of *Theory at a Glance*. I am especially impressed that the lead authors, Dr. Barbara K. Rimer and Dr. Karen Glanz, have enhanced and updated it throughout without diminishing the clarity and efficiency of the original. We hope that this new edition will empower another generation of public health practitioners to apply the same conceptual rigor to program planning and design that these authors exemplify in their own research and practice.

Robert T. Croyle, Ph.D.
Director
Division of Cancer Control and Population Sciences
National Cancer Institute

Spring 2005

Acknowledgements

The National Cancer Institute would like to thank Barbara Rimer Dr.P.H. and Karen Glanz Ph.D., M.P.H., authors of the original monograph, whose knowledge of healthcommunications theory and practice have molded a generation of health promotion practitioners. Both have provided hours of review and consultation, and we are grateful to them for their contributions.

Thanks to the staffs of the Office of Communications, particularly Margaret Farrell, and the Division of Cancer Control and Population Sciences and Kelly Blake, who guided this monograph to completion. We appreciate in particular the work of Karen Harris, whose attention to detail and commitment to excellence enhanced the monograph's content and quality.

Table of Contents

Introduction	viii
Audience and Purpose	1
Contents	1
Part 1: Foundations of Theory in Health Promotion and Health Behavior	**3**
Why Is Theory Important to Health Promotion and Health Behavior Practice?	4
What Is Theory?	4
How Can Theory Help Plan Effective Programs?	4
Explanatory Theory and Change Theory	5
Fitting Theory to the Field of Practice	5
Using Theory to Address Health Issues in Diverse Populations	7
Part 2: Theories and Applications	**9**
The Ecological Perspective: A Multilevel, Interactive Approach	10
Theoretical Explanations of Three Levels of Influence	12
Individual or Intrapersonal Level	12
Health Belief Model	13
Stages of Change Model	15
Theory of Planned Behavior	16
Precaution Adoption Process Model	18
Interpersonal Level	19
Social Cognitive Theory	19
Community Level	22
Community Organization and Other Participatory Models	23
Diffusion of Innovations	27
Communication Theory	29
Media Effects	30
Agenda Setting	30
New Communication Technologies	31
Part 3: Putting Theory and Practice Together	**35**
Planning Models	36
Social Marketing	36
PRECEDE-PROCEED	39
Where to Begin: Choosing the Right Theories	43
A Few Final Words	44
Sources	48
References	49

Tables and Figures

Tables

Table 1	An Ecological Perspective: Levels of Influence	11
Table 2	Health Belief Model	14
Table 3	Stages of Change Model	15
Table 4	Theory of Planned Behavior	17
Table 5	Social Cognitive Theory	20
Table 6	Community Organization	24
Table 7	Concepts in Diffusion of Innovations	27
Table 8	Key Attributes Affecting the Speed and Extent of an Innovation's Diffusion	28
Table 9	Agenda Setting, Concepts, Definitions, and Applications	31
Table 10	Diagnostic Elements of PRECEDE-PROCEED	42
Table 11	Summary of Theories: Focus and Key Concepts	45

Figures

Figure 1	Using Explanatory Theory and Change Theory to Plan and Evaluate Programs	6
Figure 2	A Multilevel Approach to Epidemiology	10
Figure 3	Theory of Reasoned Action and Theory of Planned Behavior	18
Figure 4	Stages of the Precaution Adoption Process Model	19
Figure 5	An Integrative Model	21
Figure 6	Sociocultural Environment Logic Framework	26
Figure 7	An Asthma Self-Management Video Game for Children	33
Figure 8	Social Marketing Wheel	38
Figure 9	The PRECEDE-PROCEED Model	40
Figure 10	Using Theory to Plan Multilevel Interventions	46

Introduction

This monograph, *Theory at a Glance: Application to Health Promotion and Health Behavior (Second Edition)*, describes influential theories of health-related behaviors, processes of shaping behavior, and the effects of community and environmental factors on behavior. It complements existing resources that offer tools, techniques, and model programs for practice, such as *Making Health Communication Programs Work: A Planner's Guide*,[i] and the Web portal, Cancer Control PLANET (Plan, Link, Act, Network with Evidence-based Tools).[ii] *Theory at a Glance* makes health behavior theory accessible and provides tools to solve problems and assess the effectiveness of health promotion programs. (For the purposes of this monograph, *health promotion* is broadly defined as the process of enabling people to increase control over, and to improve, their health. Thus, the focus goes beyond traditional primary and secondary prevention programs.)

For nearly a decade, public health and health care practitioners have consulted the original version of *Theory at a Glance* for guidance on using theories about human behavior to inform program planning, implementation, and evaluation. We have received many testimonials about the First Edition's usefulness, and requests for additional copies. This updated edition includes information from recent health behavior research and suggests theoretical approaches to developing programs for diverse populations. *Theory at a Glance* can be used as a stand-alone handbook, as part of in-house staff development programs, or in conjunction with theory texts and continuing education workshops.

For easy reference, the monograph includes only a small number of current and applicable health behavior theories. The theories reviewed here are widely used for the purposes of cancer control, defining risk, and segmenting populations. Much of the content for this publication has been adapted from the third edition of Glanz, Rimer, and Lewis' *Health Behavior and Health Education: Theory, Research, and Practice*,[1] published by Jossey-Bass in San Francisco. Readers who want to learn more about useful theories for health behavior change and health education practice can consult this and other sources that are recommended in the References section at the end of the monograph.

---

[i] *Making Health Communication Programs Work (http://www.nci.nih.gov/pinkbook/) describes a practical approach for planning and implementing health communication efforts.*

[ii] *Cancer Control PLANET (http://cancercontrolplanet.cancer.gov) provides access to data and resources that can help planners, program staff, and researchers to design, implement, and evaluate evidence-based cancer control programs.*

■ Audience and Purpose

This monograph is written primarily for public health workers in state and local health agencies; it is also valuable for health promotion practitioners and volunteers who work in voluntary health agencies, community organizations, health care settings, schools, and the private sector.

Interventions based on health behavior theory are not guaranteed to succeed, but they are much more likely to produce desired outcomes. *Theory at a Glance* is designed to help users understand how individuals, groups, and organizations behave and change—knowledge they can use to design effective programs. For information about specific, evidence-based interventions to promote health and prevent disease, readers may also wish to consult the Guide to Community Preventive Services, published by the Centers for Disease Control and Prevention (CDC) at www.thecommunityguide.org.

■ Contents

This monograph consists of three parts. For each theory, the text highlights key concepts and their applications. These summaries may be used as "checklists" of important issues to consider when planning or evaluating programs or to prompt project teams to think about the range of factors that influence health behavior.

Part 1. Foundations of Theory in Health Promotion and Health Behavior describes ways that theories and models can be useful in health behavior/health promotion practice and provides basic definitions.

Part 2. Theories and Applications presents an ecological perspective on health behavior/health promotion programs. It describes eight theories and models that explain individual, interpersonal, and community behavior and offers approaches to solving problems. A brief description of each theory is followed by definitions of key concepts and examples or case studies. The section also explores the use of new communication technologies.

Part 3. Putting Theory and Practice Together explains how theory can be used in health behavior/health promotion program planning, implementation, and evaluation. Two comprehensive planning models, PRECEDE-PROCEED and social marketing, are reviewed.

Part 1

Foundations of Theory in Health Promotion and Health Behavior

Why Is Theory Important to Health Promotion and Health Behavior Practice?

Effective public health, health promotion, and chronic disease management programs help people maintain and improve health, reduce disease risks, and manage chronic illness. They can improve the well-being and self-sufficiency of individuals, families, organizations, and communities. Usually, such successes require behavior change at many levels, (e.g., individual, organizational, and community).

Not all health programs and initiatives are equally successful, however. Those most likely to achieve desired outcomes are based on a clear understanding of targeted health behaviors, and the environmental context in which they occur. Practitioners use strategic planning models to develop and manage these programs, and continually improve them through meaningful evaluation. Health behavior theory can play a critical role throughout the program planning process.

What Is Theory?

A theory presents a systematic way of understanding events or situations. It is a set of concepts, definitions, and propositions that explain or predict these events or situations by illustrating the relationships between variables. Theories must be applicable to a broad variety of situations. They are, by nature, abstract, and don't have a specified content or topic area. Like empty coffee cups, theories have shapes and boundaries, but nothing inside. They become useful when filled with practical topics, goals, and problems.

- *Concepts* are the building blocks—the primary elements—of a theory.
- *Constructs* are concepts developed or adopted for use in a particular theory. The key concepts of a given theory are its constructs.
- *Variables* are the operational forms of constructs. They define the way a construct is to be measured in a specific situation. Match variables to constructs when identifying what needs to be assessed during evaluation of a theory-driven program.
- *Models* may draw on a number of theories to help understand a particular problem in a certain setting or context. They are not always as specified as theory.

Most health behavior and health promotion theories were adapted from the social and behavioral sciences, but applying them to health issues often requires that one be familiar with epidemiology and the biological sciences. Health behavior and health promotion theories draw upon various disciplines, such as psychology, sociology, anthropology, consumer behavior, and marketing. Many are not highly developed or have not been rigorously tested. Because of this, they often are called *conceptual frameworks* or *theoretical frameworks*; here the terms are used interchangeably.

How Can Theory Help Plan Effective Programs?

Theory gives planners tools for moving beyond intuition to design and evaluate health behavior and health promotion interventions based on understanding of behavior. It helps them to step back and consider the larger picture. Like an artist, a program planner who grounds health interventions in theory creates innovative ways to address specific circumstances. He or she does not depend on a "paint-by-numbers" approach, re-hashing stale ideas, but uses a palette of behavior theories, skillfully applying them to develop unique, tailored solutions to problems.

Using theory as a foundation for program planning and development is consistent with the current emphasis on using evidence-based interventions in public health, behavioral medicine, and medicine. Theory provides a road map for studying problems, developing appropriate interventions, and evaluating their successes. It can inform the planner's thinking during all of these stages, offering insights that translate into stronger programs. Theory can also help to explain the dynamics of health behaviors, including processes for changing them, and the influences of the many forces that affect health behaviors, including social and physical environments. Theory can also help planners identify the most suitable target audiences, methods for fostering change, and outcomes for evaluation.

Researchers and practitioners use theory to investigate answers to the questions of "why," "what," and "how" health problems should be addressed. By seeking answers to these questions, they clarify the nature of targeted health behaviors. That is, theory guides the search for reasons why people do or do not engage in certain health behaviors; it helps pinpoint what planners need to know before they develop public health programs; and it suggests how to devise program strategies that reach target audiences and have an impact. Theory also helps to identify which indicators should be monitored and measured during program evaluation. For these reasons, program planning, implementation, and monitoring processes based in theory are more likely to succeed than those developed without the benefit of a theoretical perspective.

Explanatory Theory and Change Theory

Explanatory theory describes the reasons why a problem exists. It guides the search for factors that contribute to a problem (e.g., a lack of knowledge, self-efficacy, social support, or resources), and can be changed. Examples of explanatory theories include the Health Belief Model, the Theory of Planned Behavior, and the Precaution Adoption Process Model.

Change theory guides the development of health interventions. It spells out concepts that can be translated into program messages and strategies, and offers a basis for program evaluation. Change theory helps program planners to be explicit about their assumptions for why a program will work. Examples of change theories include Community Organization and Diffusion of Innovations. Figure 1. illustrates how explanatory theory and change theory can be used to plan and evaluate programs.

Fitting Theory to the Field of Practice

This monograph includes descriptions and applications of some theories that are central to health behavior and health promotion practice today. No single theory dominates health education and promotion, nor should it; the problems, behaviors, populations, cultures, and contexts of public health practice are broad and varied. Some theories focus on individuals as the unit of change. Others examine change within families, institutions, communities, or cultures. Adequately addressing an issue may require more than one theory, and no one theory is suitable for all cases.

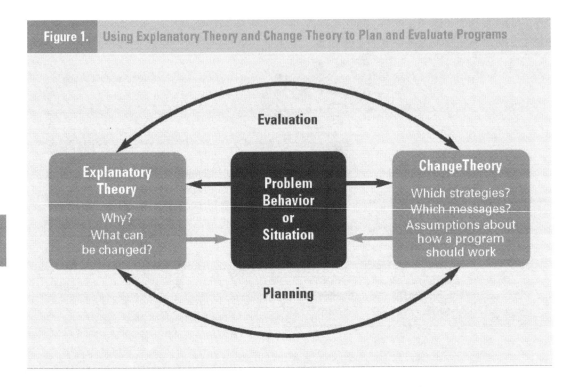

Figure 1. Using Explanatory Theory and Change Theory to Plan and Evaluate Programs

Because the social context in which behavior occurs is always evolving, theories that were important in public health education a generation ago may be of limited use today. At the same time, new social science research allows theorists to refine and adapt existing theories. A recent Institute of Medicine report[2] observed that several theorists have converged in their views, identifying several variables as central to behavior change. As a result, some constructs, such as self-efficacy, are central to multiple theories.

Effective practice depends on using theories and strategies that are appropriate to a situation.

One of the greatest challenges for those concerned with behavior change is learning to analyze how well a theory or model "fits" a particular issue. A working knowledge of specific theories, and familiarity with how they have been applied in the past, improves skills in this area. Selecting an appropriate theory or combination of theories helps take into account the multiple factors that influence health behaviors. The practitioner who uses theory develops a nuanced understanding of realistic program outcomes that drives the planning process.

Choosing a theory that will bring a useful perspective to the problem at hand does not begin with a theory (e.g., the most familiar theory, the theory mentioned in a recent journal article, etc.). Instead, this process starts with a thorough assessment of the situation: the units of analysis or change, the topic, and the type of behavior to be addressed. Because different theoretical frameworks are appropriate and practical for different situations, selecting a theory that "fits" should be a careful, deliberate process. Start with the steps in the box at the top of the next page.

A Good Fit: Characteristics of a Useful Theory

A useful theory makes assumptions about a behavior, health problem, target population, or environment that are:

- Logical;
- Consistent with everyday observations;
- Similar to those used in previous successful programs; and
- Supported by past research in the same area or related ideas.

Using Theory to Address Health Issues in Diverse Populations

The U.S. population is growing more culturally and ethnically diverse. An increasing body of research shows health disparities exist among various ethnic and socio-economic groups. These findings highlight the importance of understanding the cultural backgrounds and life experiences of community members, though research has not yet established when and under what circumstances targeted or tailored health communications are more effective than generic ones. (Targeting involves using information about shared characteristics of a population subgroup to create a single intervention approach for that group. In contrast, tailoring is a process that uses an assessment to derive information about one specific person, and then offers change or information strategies for an outcome of interest based on that person's unique characteristics.)[3]

Most health behavior theories can be applied to diverse cultural and ethnic groups, but health practitioners must understand the characteristics of target populations (e.g., ethnicity, socioeconomic status, gender, age, and geographical location) to use these theories correctly.

There are several reasons why culture and ethnicity are critical to consider when applying theory to a health problem. First, morbidity and mortality rates for different diseases vary by race and ethnicity; second, there are differences in the prevalence of risk behaviors among these groups; and third, the determinants of health behaviors vary across racial and ethnic groups.

What People in the Field Say About Theory

"Theory is different from most of the tools I use in my work. It's more abstract, but that can be a plus too. A solid grounding in a handful of theories goes a long way toward helping me think through why I approach a health problem the way I do."

— *County Health Educator*

"I used to think theory was just for students and researchers. But now I have a better grasp of it; I appreciate how practical it can be."

— *State Chronic Disease Administrator*

"By translating concepts from theory into real-world terms, I can get my staff and community volunteers to take a closer look at <u>why</u> we're conducting programs the way we do, and <u>how</u> they can succeed or fail."

— *City Tobacco Control Coordinator*

"A good grasp of theory is essential for leadership. It gives you a broader way of viewing your work. And it helps create a vision for the future. But, of course, it's only worthwhile if I can translate it clearly and simply to my co-workers."

— *Regional Health Promotion Chief*

"It's not as hard as I thought it would be to keep up with current theories. More than ever these days, there are tools and workshops to update us often."

— *Patient Education Coordinator*

Part 2

Theories and Applications

PART 2

9 — THEORY AT A GLANCE

The Ecological Perspective: A Multilevel, Interactive Approach

Contemporary health promotion involves more than simply educating individuals about healthy practices. It includes efforts to change organizational behavior, as well as the physical and social environment of communities. It is also about developing and advocating for policies that support health, such as economic incentives. Health promotion programs that seek to address health problems across this spectrum employ a range of strategies, and operate on multiple levels.

The *ecological perspective* emphasizes the interaction between, and interdependence of, factors within and across all levels of a health problem. It highlights people's interactions with their physical and socio-cultural environments. Two key concepts of the ecological perspective help to identify intervention points for promoting health: first, behavior both affects, and is affected by, *multiple levels of influence*; second, individual behavior both shapes, and is shaped by, the social environment (*reciprocal causation*).

To explain the first key concept of the ecological perspective, multiple levels of influence, McLeroy and colleagues (1988)[4] identified five levels of influence for health-related behaviors and conditions. Defined in Table 1., these levels include: (1) *intrapersonal* or *individual* factors; (2) *interpersonal* factors; (3) *institutional* or *organizational* factors; (4) *community* factors; and (5) *public policy* factors.

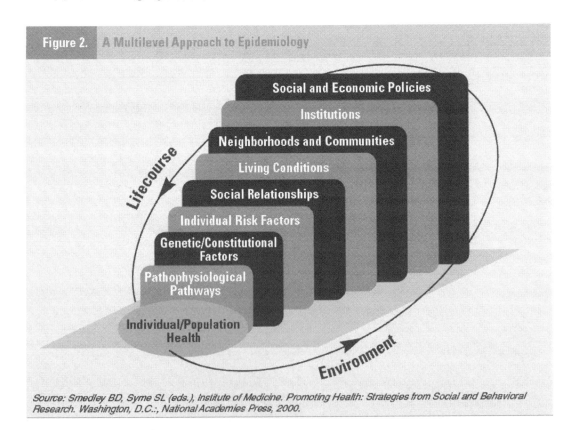

Figure 2. A Multilevel Approach to Epidemiology

Source: Smedley BD, Syme SL (eds.), Institute of Medicine. *Promoting Health: Strategies from Social and Behavioral Research.* Washington, D.C.: National Academies Press, 2000.

Table 1. An Ecological Perspective: Levels of Influence

Concept	Definition
Intrapersonal Level	Individual characteristics that influence behavior, such as knowledge, attitudes, beliefs, and personality traits
Interpersonal Level	Interpersonal processes and primary groups, including family, friends, and peers that provide social identity, support, and role definition
Community Level Institutional Factors	Rules, regulations, policies, and informal structures, which may constrain or promote recommended behaviors
Community Factors	Social networks and norms, or standards, which exist as formal or informal among individuals, groups, and organizations
Public Policy	Local, state, and federal policies and laws that regulate or support healthy actions and practices for disease prevention, early detection, control, and management

In practice, addressing the community level requires taking into consideration institutional and public policy factors, as well as social networks and norms. Figure 2. illustrates how different levels of influence combine to affect population health.

Each level of influence can affect health behavior. For example, suppose a woman delays getting a recommended mammogram (screening for breast cancer). At the individual level, her inaction may be due to fears of finding out she has cancer.

At the interpersonal level, her doctor may neglect to tell her that she should get the test, or she may have friends who say they do not believe it is important to get a mammogram. At the organizational level, it may be hard to schedule an appointment, because there is only a part-time radiologist at the clinic. At the policy level, she may lack insurance coverage, and thus be unable to afford the fee. Thus, the outcome, the woman's failure to get a mammogram, may result from multiple factors.

The second key concept of an ecological perspective, reciprocal causation, suggests that people both influence, and are influenced by, those around them. For example, a man with high cholesterol may find it hard to follow the diet his doctor has prescribed because his company cafeteria doesn't offer healthy food choices. To comply with his doctor's instructions, he can try to change the environment by asking the cafeteria manager to add healthy items to the menu, or he can dine elsewhere. If he and enough of his fellow employees decide to find someplace else to eat, the cafeteria may change its menu to maintain lunch business. Thus, the cafeteria environment may compel this man to change his dining habits, but his new habits may ultimately bring about change in the cafeteria as well.

An ecological perspective shows the advantages of multilevel interventions that combine behavioral and environmental components. For instance, effective tobacco control programs often use multiple strategies to discourage smoking.[5] Employee smoking cessation clinics have a stronger impact if the workplace has a no-smoking policy and the city has a clean indoor air ordinance. Adolescents are less likely to begin smoking if their peers disapprove of the habit and laws prohibiting tobacco sales to minors are strictly enforced. Health promotion programs are more effective when planners consider multiple levels of influence on health problems.

Theoretical Explanations of Three Levels of Influence

The next three sections examine theories and their applications at the individual (intrapersonal), interpersonal, and community levels of the ecological perspective. At the individual and interpersonal levels, contemporary theories of health behavior can be broadly categorized as "Cognitive-Behavioral." Three key concepts cut across these theories:

1. Behavior is mediated by cognitions; that is, what people know and think affects how they act.

2. Knowledge is necessary for, but not sufficient to produce, most behavior changes.

3. Perceptions, motivations, skills, and the social environment are key influences on behavior.

Community-level models offer frameworks for implementing multi-dimensional approaches to promote healthy behaviors. They supplement educational approaches with efforts to change the social and physical environment to support positive behavior change.

Individual or Intrapersonal Level

The individual level is the most basic one in health promotion practice, so planners must be able to explain and influence the behavior of individuals. Many health practitioners spend most of their work time in one-on-one activities such as counseling or patient education, and individuals are often the primary target audience for health education materials. Because individual behavior is the fundamental unit of group behavior, individual-level behavior change theories often comprise broader-level models of group, organizational, community, and national behavior. Individuals participate in groups, manage organizations, elect and appoint leaders, and legislate policy. Thus, achieving policy and institutional change requires influencing individuals.

In addition to exploring behavior, individual-level theories focus on intrapersonal factors (those existing or occurring within the individual self or mind). Intrapersonal factors include knowledge, attitudes, beliefs, motivation, self-concept, developmental history, past experience, and skills. Individual-level theories are presented below.

- *The Health Belief Model (HBM)* addresses the individual's perceptions of the threat posed by a health problem (susceptibility, severity), the benefits of avoiding the threat, and factors influencing the decision to act (barriers, cues to action, and self-efficacy).

- *The Stages of Change (Transtheoretical) Model* describes individuals' motivation and readiness to change a behavior.

- *The Theory of Planned Behavior (TPB)* examines the relations between an individual's beliefs, attitudes, intentions, behavior, and perceived control over that behavior.

- *The Precaution Adoption Process Model (PAPM)* names seven stages in an individual's journey from awareness to action. It begins with lack of awareness and advances through subsequent stages of becoming aware, deciding whether or not to act, acting, and maintaining the behavior.

Health Belief Model (HBM)

The Health Belief Model (HBM) was one of the first theories of health behavior, and remains one of the most widely recognized in the field. It was developed in the 1950s by a group of U.S. Public Health Service social psychologists who wanted to explain why so few people were participating in programs to prevent and detect disease. For example, the Public Health Service was sending mobile X-ray units out to neighborhoods to offer free chest X-rays (screening for tuberculosis). Despite the fact that this service was offered without charge in a variety of convenient locations, the program was of limited success. The question was, "Why?"

To find an answer, social psychologists examined what was encouraging or discouraging people from participating in the programs. They theorized that people's beliefs about whether or not they were susceptible to disease, and their perceptions of the benefits of trying to avoid it, influenced their readiness to act.

In ensuing years, researchers expanded upon this theory, eventually concluding that six main constructs influence people's decisions about whether to take action to prevent, screen for, and control illness. They argued that people are ready to act if they:

- Believe they are susceptible to the condition (*perceived susceptibility*)

- Believe the condition has serious consequences (*perceived severity*)

- Believe taking action would reduce their susceptibility to the condition or its severity (*perceived benefits*)

- Believe costs of taking action (*perceived barriers*) are outweighed by the benefits

- Are exposed to factors that prompt action (e.g., a television ad or a reminder from one's physician to get a mammogram) (*cue to action*)

- Are confident in their ability to successfully perform an action (*self-efficacy*)

Since health motivation is its central focus, the HBM is a good fit for addressing problem behaviors that evoke health concerns (e.g., high-risk sexual behavior and the possibility of contracting HIV). Together, the six constructs of the HBM provide a useful framework for designing both short-term and long-term behavior change strategies. (See Table 2.) When applying the HBM to planning health programs, practitioners should ground their efforts in an understanding of how susceptible the target population feels to the health problem, whether they believe it is serious, and whether they believe action can reduce the threat at an acceptable cost. Attempting to effect changes in these factors is rarely as simple as it may appear.

Table 2. Health Belief Model

Concept	Definition	Potential Change Strategies
Perceived susceptibility	Beliefs about the chances of getting a condition	• Define what populations(s) are at risk and their levels of risk • Tailor risk information based on an individual's characteristics or behaviors • Help the individual develop an accurate perception of his or her own risk
Perceived severity	Beliefs about the seriousness of a condition and its consequences	• Specify the consequences of a condition and recommended action
Perceived benefits	Beliefs about the effectiveness of taking action to reduce risk or seriousness	• Explain how, where, and when to take action and what the potential positive results will be
Perceived barriers	Beliefs about the material and psychological costs of taking action	• Offer reassurance, incentives, and assistance; correct misinformation
Cues to action	Factors that activate "readiness to change"	• Provide "how to" information, promote awareness, and employ reminder systems
Self-efficacy	Confidence in one's ability to take action	• Provide training and guidance in performing action • Use progressive goal setting • Give verbal reinforcement • Demonstrate desired behaviors

High blood pressure screening campaigns often identify people who are at high risk for heart disease and stroke, but who say they have not experienced any symptoms. Because they don't feel sick, they may not follow instructions to take prescribed medicine or lose weight. The HBM can be useful for developing strategies to deal with noncompliance in such situations.

According to the HBM, asymptomatic people may not follow a prescribed treatment regimen unless they accept that, though they have no symptoms, they do in fact have hypertension (perceived susceptibility). They must understand that hypertension can lead to heart attacks and strokes (perceived severity). Taking prescribed medication or following a recommended weight loss program will reduce the risks (perceived benefits) without negative side effects or excessive difficulty (perceived barriers). Print materials, reminder letters, or pill calendars might encourage people to consistently follow their doctors' recommendations (cues to action). For those who have, in the past, had a hard time losing weight or maintaining weight loss, a behavioral contract might help establish achievable, short-term goals to build confidence (self-efficacy).

Stages of Change (Transtheoretical) Model
Developed by Prochaska and DiClemente,[6] the Stages of Change Model evolved out of studies comparing the experiences of smokers who quit on their own with those of smokers receiving professional treatment. The model's basic premise is that behavior change is a process, not an event. As a person attempts to change a behavior, he or she moves through five stages: *precontemplation, contemplation, preparation, action,* and *maintenance* (see Table 3.). Definitions of the stages vary slightly, depending on the behavior at issue. People at different points along this continuum have different informational needs, and benefit from interventions designed for their stage.

Whether individuals use self-management methods or take part in professional programs, they go through the same stages of change. Nonetheless, the manner in which they pass through these stages may vary, depending on the type of behavior change. For example, a person who is trying to give up smoking may experience the stages differently than someone who is seeking to improve their dietary habits by eating more fruits and vegetables.

The Stages of Change Model has been applied to a variety of individual behaviors, as well as to organizational change. The Model is circular, not linear. In other words, people do not systematically progress from one stage to the next, ultimately "graduating" from the behavior change process. Instead, they may enter the change process at any stage, relapse to an earlier stage, and begin the process once more. They may cycle through this process repeatedly, and the process can truncate at any point.

Table 3. Stages of Change Model

Stage	Definition	Potential Change Strategies
Precontemplation	Has no intention of taking action within the next six months	Increase awareness of need for change; personalize information about risks and benefits
Contemplation	Intends to take action in the next six months	Motivate; encourage making specific plans
Preparation	Intends to take action within the next thirty days and has taken some behavioral steps in this direction	Assist with developing and implementing concrete action plans; help set gradual goals
Action	Has changed behavior for less than six months	Assist with feedback, problem solving, social support, and reinforcement
Maintenance	Has changed behavior for more than six months	Assist with coping, reminders, finding alternatives, avoiding slips/relapses (as applicable)

> Suppose a large company hires a health educator to plan a smoking cessation program for its employees who smoke (200 people). The health educator decides to offer group smoking cessation clinics to employees at various times and locations. Several months pass, however, and only 50 of the smokers sign up for the clinics. At this point, the health educator faces a dilemma: how can the 150 smokers who are not participating in the clinics be reached?
>
> The Stages of Change Model offers perspective on ways to approach this problem. First, the model can be employed to help understand and explain why they are not attending the clinics. Second, it can be used to develop a comprehensive smoking program to help more current and former smokers change their smoking behavior, and maintain that change. By asking a few simple questions, the health educator can assess what stages of contemplation potential program participants are in. For example:
>
> - Are you interested in trying to quit smoking? (Pre-contemplation)
> - Are you thinking about quitting smoking soon? (Contemplation)
> - Are you ready to plan how you will quit smoking? (Preparation)
> - Are you in the process of trying to quit smoking? (Action)
> - Are you trying to stay smoke-free? (Maintenance)
>
> The employees' responses will help to pinpoint where the participants are on the continuum of change, and to tailor messages, strategies, and programs appropriate to their needs. For example, individuals who enjoy smoking are not interested in trying to quit, and therefore will not attend a smoking cessation clinic; for them, a more appropriate intervention might include educational interventions designed to move them out of the "precontemplation" stage and into "contemplation" (e.g., using carbon monoxide testing to demonstrate the effect of smoking on health). On the other hand, individuals who are ready to plan how to quit smoking (the "preparation" stage) can be encouraged to do so, and moved to the next stage, "action."

Theory of Planned Behavior (TPB)

The Theory of Planned Behavior (TPB) and the associated Theory of Reasoned Action (TRA) explore the relationship between behavior and beliefs, attitudes, and intentions. Both the TPB and the TRA assume *behavioral intention* is the most important determinant of behavior. According to these models, behavioral intention is influenced by a person's *attitude* toward performing a behavior, and by beliefs about whether individuals who are important to the person approve or disapprove of the behavior (*subjective norm*). The TPB and TRA assume all other factors (e.g., culture, the environment) operate through the models' constructs, and do not independently explain the likelihood that a person will behave a certain way.

The TPB differs from the TRA in that it includes one additional construct, *perceived behavioral control*; this construct has to do with people's beliefs that they can control a particular behavior. Azjen and Driver[7] added this construct to account for situations in which people's behavior, or behavioral intention, is influenced by factors beyond their control. They argued that people might try harder to perform a behavior if they feel they have a high degree of control over it. (See Table 4.) It has application beyond these limited situations, however. People's perceptions about controllability may have an important influence on behavior.

Table 4. Theory of Planned Behavior

Concept	Definition	Measurement Approach
Behavioral intention	Perceived likelihood of performing behavior	Are you likely or unlikely to (perform the behavior)?
Attitude	Personal evaluation of the behavior	Do you see (the behavior) as good, neutral, or bad?
Subjective norm	Beliefs about whether key people approve or disapprove of the behavior; motivation to behave in a way that gains their approval	Do you agree or disagree that most people approve of/disapprove of (the behavior)?
Perceived behavioral control	Belief that one has, and can exercise, control over performing the behavior	Do you believe (performing the behavior) is up to you, or not up to you?

Surveillance data show that young, acculturated Hispanic women are more likely to get Pap tests than those who are older and less acculturated.[8] A health department decides to implement a cervical cancer screening program targeting older Hispanic women. In planning the campaign, practitioners want to conduct a survey to learn what beliefs, attitudes, and intentions in this population are associated with seeking a Pap test. They design the survey to gauge: when the women received their last Pap test (behavior); how likely they are to seek a Pap test (intention); attitudes about getting a Pap test (attitude); whether or not "most people who are important to me" would want them to get a Pap test (subjective norm); and whether or not getting a Pap test is something that is "under my control" (perceived behavioral control). The department will compare survey results with data about who has or has not received a Pap test to identify beliefs, attitudes, and intentions that predict seeking one.

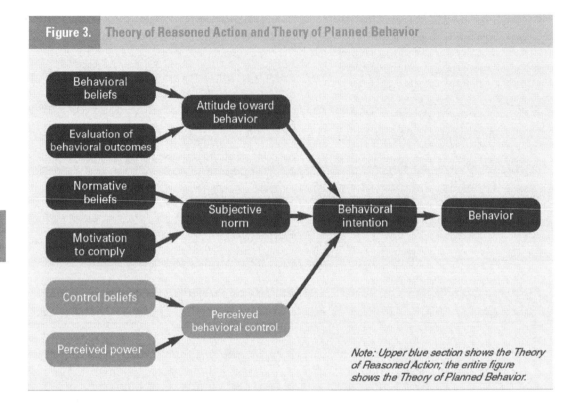

Note: Upper blue section shows the Theory of Reasoned Action; the entire figure shows the Theory of Planned Behavior.

Figure 3. shows the TPB's explanation for how *behavioral intention* determines *behavior*, and how *attitude toward behavior*, *subjective norm*, and *perceived behavioral control* influence *behavioral intention*. According to the model, attitudes toward behavior are shaped by beliefs about what is entailed in performing the behavior and outcomes of the behavior. Beliefs about social standards and motivation to comply with those norms affect *subjective norms*. The presence or lack of things that will make it easier or harder to perform the behavior affect *perceived behavioral control*. Thus, a causal chain of beliefs, attitudes, and intentions drives *behavior*.

Precaution Adoption Process Model
The Precaution Adoption Process Model (PAPM) specifies seven distinct stages in the journey from lack of awareness to adoption and/or maintenance of a behavior. It is a relatively new model that has been applied to an increasing number of health behaviors, including: osteoporosis prevention, colorectal cancer screening, mammography, hepatitis B vaccination, and home testing for radon gas.

In the first stage of the PAPM, an individual may be completely unaware of a hazard (e.g., radon exposure, the link between unprotected sex and HIV). The person may subsequently become aware of the issue but remain unengaged by it (Stage 2). Next, the person faces a decision about acting (Stage 3); may decide not to act (Stage 4),

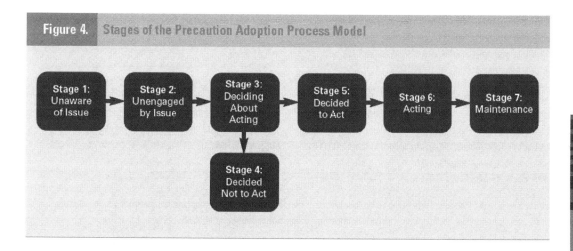

Figure 4. Stages of the Precaution Adoption Process Model

or may decide to act (Stage 5). The stages of action (Stage 6) and maintenance (Stage 7) follow. (See Figure 4.) According to the PAPM, people pass through each stage of precaution adoption without skipping any of them. It is possible for people to move backwards from some later stages to earlier ones, but once they have completed the first two stages of the model they do not return to them. For example, a person does not move from unawareness to awareness and then back to unawareness.

The PAPM bears similarities to the Stages of Change model, but differs in important ways. Stages of Change offers insights for addressing hard-to-change behaviors such as smoking or overeating; it is less helpful when dealing with hazards that have recently been recognized or precautions that are newly available. The PAPM recognizes that people who are unaware of an issue, or are unengaged by it, face different barriers from those who have decided not to act. The PAPM prompts practitioners to develop intervention strategies that take into account the stages that precede active decision-making.

Interpersonal Level

At the interpersonal level, theories of health behavior assume individuals exist within, and are influenced by, a social environment. The opinions, thoughts, behavior, advice, and support of the people surrounding an individual influence his or her feelings and behavior, and the individual has a reciprocal effect on those people. The social environment includes family members, coworkers, friends, health professionals, and others. Because it affects behavior, the social environment also impacts health. Many theories focus at the interpersonal level, but this monograph highlights Social Cognitive Theory (SCT). SCT is one of the most frequently used and robust health behavior theories. It explores the reciprocal interactions of people and their environments, and the psychosocial determinants of health behavior.

Social Cognitive Theory (SCT)

Social Cognitive Theory (SCT) describes a dynamic, ongoing process in which personal factors, environmental factors, and human behavior exert influence upon each other.

According to SCT, three main factors affect the likelihood that a person will change a health behavior: (1) self-efficacy, (2) goals, and (3) outcome expectancies. If individuals have a sense of personal agency or self-efficacy, they can change behaviors even when faced with obstacles. If they do not feel that they can exercise control over their health behavior, they are not motivated to act, or to persist through challenges.[9] As a person adopts new behaviors, this causes changes in both the environment and in the person. Behavior is not simply a product of the environment and the person, and environment is not simply a product of the person and behavior.

SCT evolved from research on Social Learning Theory (SLT), which asserts that people learn not only from their own experiences, but by observing the actions of others and the benefits of those actions. Bandura updated SLT, adding the construct of self-efficacy and renaming it SCT. (Though SCT is the dominant version in current practice, it is still sometimes called SLT.) SCT integrates concepts and processes from cognitive, behaviorist, and emotional models of behavior change, so it includes many constructs. (See Table 5.) It has been used successfully as the underlying theory for behavior change in areas ranging from dietary change[10] to pain control.[11]

Table 5. Social Cognitive Theory

Concept	Definition	Potential Change Strategies
Reciprocal determinism	The dynamic interaction of the person, behavior, and the environment in which the behavior is performed	Consider multiple ways to promote behavior change, including making adjustments to the environment or influencing personal attitudes
Behavioral capability	Knowledge and skill to perform a given behavior	Promote mastery learning through skills training
Expectations	Anticipated outcomes of a behavior	Model positive outcomes of healthful behavior
Self-efficacy	Confidence in one's ability to take action and overcome barriers	Approach behavior change in small steps to ensure success; be specific about the desired change
Observational learning (modeling)	Behavioral acquisition that occurs by watching the actions and outcomes of others' behavior	Offer credible role models who perform the targeted behavior
Reinforcements	Responses to a person's behavior that increase or decrease the likelihood of reoccurrence	Promote self-initiated rewards and incentives

Reciprocal determinism describes interactions between behavior, personal factors, and environment, where each influences the others. *Behavioral capability* states that, to perform a behavior, a person must know what to do and how to do it. *Expectations* are the results an individual anticipates from taking action. Bandura considers *self-efficacy* the most important personal factor in behavior change, and it is a nearly ubiquitous construct in health behavior theories. Strategies for increasing self-efficacy include: setting incremental goals (e.g., exercising for 10 minutes each day); behavioral contracting (a formal contract, with specified goals and rewards); and monitoring and reinforcement (feedback from self-monitoring or record keeping).

Observational learning, or *modeling*, refers to the process whereby people learn through the experiences of credible others, rather than through their own experience. *Reinforcements* are responses to behavior that affect whether or not one will repeat it. Positive reinforcements (rewards) increase a person's likelihood of repeating the behavior. Negative reinforcements may make repeated behavior more likely by motivating the person to eliminate a negative stimulus (e.g., when drivers put the key in the car's ignition, the beeping alarm reminds them to fasten their seatbelt). Reinforcements can be *internal* or *external.* Internal rewards are things people do to reward themselves. External rewards (e.g., token incentives) encourage continued participation in multiple-session programs, but generally are not effective for sustaining long-term change because they do not bolster a person's own desire or commitment to change. Figure 5. illustrates how self-efficacy, environmental, and individual factors impact behavior.

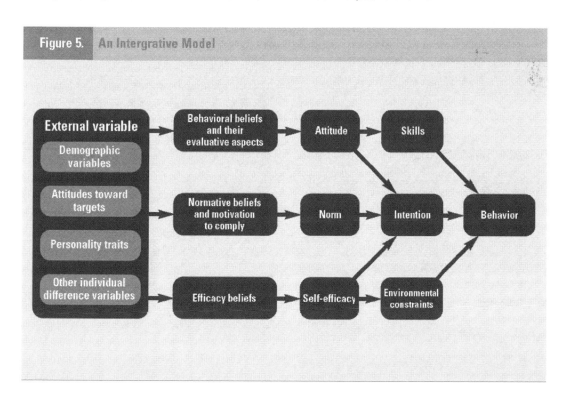

Figure 5. An Intergrative Model

> A university in a rural area develops a church-based intervention to help congregation members change their habits to meet cancer risk reduction guidelines (behavior). Many members of the church have low incomes, are overweight, rarely exercise, eat foods that are high in sugar and fat, and are uninsured (personal factors). Because of their rural location, they often must drive long distances to attend church, visit health clinics, or buy groceries (environment).
>
> The program offers classes that teach healthy cooking and exercise skills (behavioral capability). Participants learn how eating a healthy diet and exercising will benefit them (expectations). Health advisors create contracts with participants, setting incremental goals (self-efficacy). Respected congregation members serve as role models (observational learning). Participants receive T-shirts, recipe books, and other incentives, and are taught to reward themselves by making time to relax (reinforcement). As church members learn about healthy lifestyles, they bring healthier foods to church, reinforcing their healthy habits (reciprocal determinism).

■ Community Level

Initiatives serving communities and populations, not just individuals, are at the heart of public health approaches to preventing and controlling disease. Community-level models explore how social systems function and change and how to mobilize community members and organizations. They offer strategies that work in a variety of settings, such as health care institutions, schools, worksites, community groups, and government agencies. Embodying an ecological perspective, community-level models address individual, group, institutional, and community issues.

Communities are often understood in geographical terms, but they can be defined by other criteria too. For instance, there are communities of shared interests (e.g., the artists' community) or collective identity (e.g., the African American community). When planning community-level interventions, it is critical to learn about the community's unique characteristics. This is particularly true when addressing health issues in ethnically or culturally diverse communities.

Comprehensive health promotion programs often use advocacy techniques to help support individual behavior change with organizational and regulatory change. In recent years, innovative tools and methods for evaluation and measurement have been developed to capture the successes of community-level health promotion efforts.[12,13] Tobacco control/smoking prevention is one area where programs have been extensively evaluated. Local tobacco control initiatives typically pursue four concurrent goals: (1) raising the priority of smoking as a health concern, (2) helping community members to change smoking behavior, (3) strengthening legal and economic deterrents to smoking, and (4) reinforcing social norms that discourage smoking. This multi-level approach has been proven very effective.

The conceptual frameworks in this section offer strategies for intervening at the community level:

- *Community Organization and Other Participatory Models* emphasize community-driven approaches to assessing and solving health and social problems.

- *Diffusion of Innovations Theory* addresses how new ideas, products, and social practices spread within an organization, community, or society, or from one society to another.

- *Communication Theory* describes how different types of communication affect health behavior.

Community Organization and Other Participatory Models

Community organizing is a process through which community groups are helped to identify common problems, mobilize resources, and develop and implement strategies to reach collective goals. Strict definitions of community organizing assume that the community itself identifies the problems to address (not an outside change agent). Public health professionals often adapt the methods of community organizing to launch programs that reflect the priorities of community members, but may not be initiated by them. Community organizing projects that start with the community's priorities, rather than an externally imposed agenda, are more likely to succeed.

Community organizing is consistent with an ecological perspective in that it recognizes multiple levels of a health problem. It can be integrated with SCT-based strategies that take into account the dynamic between personal factors, environmental factors, and human behavior. Theories of *social networks* and *social support* (exploring the influence of social relationships on health decision making and behavior) can be used to adapt community organizing strategies to health education goals. *Social systems theory* (exploring how organizations in a community interact with each other and the outside world) is also useful for this purpose.

Community organizing is not a single mode of practice; it can involve different approaches to effecting change. Jack Rothman[14] produced the best-known classification of these change models, describing community organizing according to three general types: locality development, social planning, and social action. These models sometimes overlap and can be combined.

- *Locality development* (or community development) is process oriented. With the aim of developing group identity and cohesion, it focuses on building consensus and capacity.

- *Social planning* is task oriented. It stresses problem solving and usually relies heavily on expert practitioners.

- *Social action* is both process and task oriented. Its goals are to increase the community's capacity to solve problems and to achieve concrete changes that redress social injustices.

The different approaches broadly classified as community organizing share in common several concepts that are key to achieving and measuring change. (See Table 6.) *Empowerment* describes a social action process through which individuals, organizations, or communities gain confidence and skills to improve their quality of life.[15] *Community capacity* refers to

Table 6. Community Organization

Term	Definition	Potential Change Strategies
Empowerment	A social action process through which people gain mastery over their lives and their communities	Community members assume greater power, or expand their power from within, to create desired changes
Community capacity	Characteristics of a community that affect its ability to identify, mobilize around, and address problems	Community members participate actively in community life, gaining leadership skills, social networks, and access to power
Participation	Engagement of community members as equal partners; reflects the principle, "Never do for others what they can do for themselves"	Community members develop leadership skills, knowledge, and resources through their involvement
Relevance	Community organizing that "starts where the people are"	Community members create their own agenda based on felt needs, shared power, and awareness of resources
Issue selection	Identifying immediate, specific, and realizable targets for change that unify and build community strength	Community members participate in identifying issues; targets are chosen as part of a larger strategy
Critical consciousness	Awareness of social, political, and economic forces that contribute to social problems	Community members discuss the root causes of problems and plan actions to address them

characteristics of a community that allow it to identify social problems and address them (e.g., trusting relationships between neighbors, civic engagement). *Participation* in the organizing process helps community members to gain leadership and problem-solving skills. *Relevance* involves activating participants to address issues that are important to them. *Issue selection* entails pulling apart a web of interrelated problems into distinct, immediate, solvable pieces. *Critical consciousness* emphasizes helping community members to identify the root causes of social problems.

The social action model differs from other forms of community intervention in that it is grassroots based, conflict oriented, and geared to mobilizing disadvantaged people to act on their own behalf.[16] Goals vary, but typically include policy and other significant changes that participants have identified as important. Largely based on the organizing work of Saul Alinsky and the Industrial Areas Foundation,[17] this approach employs direct-action strategies as the primary means of fostering change. It focuses on building power and encouraging community members to develop their capacities as active citizens.[18]

In a social action approach to community organizing, *self-interest* is seen as the motivation for action: community members become involved when they see that it will benefit them to take action, and targeted institutions are willing to make changes when they believe it is in their self-interest to do so. Community organizing seeks to expand participants' sense of self-interest to an ever-wider sphere, from the individual or family level to their block, neighborhood, city, state, and so on.[19] Participants grow through this process, learning to take an active role in shaping the future of their communities.

Media Advocacy is an essential tactic in community organizing. It involves using the mass media strategically to advance public policies.[20] Because the media bring attention to specific issues, they set the agenda for the public and policy makers. The media often present health information in medical terms, focusing on technological breakthroughs and personal health habits. Media advocacy assumes the root of most health problems is not that people lack information, but that they lack the power to change social and economic conditions. It seeks to balance news coverage by framing issues to emphasize social, economic, and political—rather than personal and behavioral—influences on health.[21]

Responding to high rates of cancer among African Americans, a health department wishes to increase consumption of fresh fruits and vegetables in a low-income, urban neighborhood. The department surveys community members to find out why they do not eat more fruits and vegetables. They learn there are few supermarkets within easy walking distance, and residents shop at local stores that do not offer fresh, affordable produce. Many do not own cars; they must take the bus, spend money on taxis, or carry shopping bags for blocks to shop at the supermarket.

The health department contacts a community-based organization that has been working to improve neighborhood conditions, and shares the findings with them (participation). The organization's leaders invite department staff to attend a community meeting, where residents discuss why there are fewer supermarkets in low-income neighborhoods (critical consciousness). Residents say they would buy healthier, less expensive foods at the supermarket if they could get a ride home (relevance). The community organization decides to organize a campaign to convince the local supermarket to start a shuttle service (issue selection).

The health department trains residents to assess the potential cost and ridership of the shuttle service (community capacity). Residents plan an event and invite the media. They line up in front of the supermarket with shopping carts and signs, and explain both the problem and the potential solution to reporters (media advocacy). Stories appear in the local newspapers. The supermarket's management meets with community residents and tells them the market loses thousands of dollars each year due to stolen shopping carts. Residents explain that the store will have fewer shopping cart losses if they start a shuttle (self-interest). The supermarket agrees to give free rides to inner-city shoppers. Through their success, residents gain skills and confidence, and are inspired to think about other ways to strengthen their community (empowerment).

In participatory action research, the people who are being studied take an active role in some or all phases of the research. Participatory research builds an alliance between professional researchers and lay participants, and enables a dialogue between them.[22] When planning and implementing health programs, the program's beneficiaries help to direct the type of inquiry, collect and analyze data, imagine possible solutions, and evaluate the costs and benefits of each choice. They engage in a learning process, both checking and complementing expert knowledge. One example of participatory action research is the NCI's COMMIT program, which explored whether implementing an intervention through community organizations would result in a higher "quit rate" among heavy smokers than in the comparison communities.[23][24]

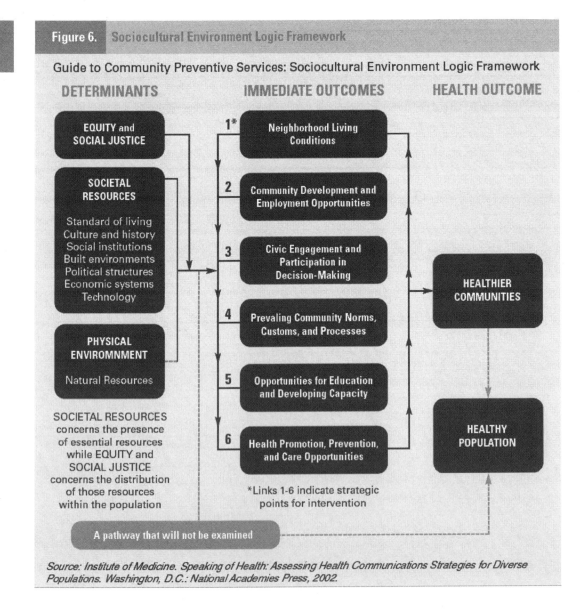

Figure 6. Sociocultural Environment Logic Framework

Source: Institute of Medicine. Speaking of Health: Assessing Health Communications Strategies for Diverse Populations. Washington, D.C.: National Academies Press, 2002.

The CDC Task Force on the *Guide to Community and Preventive Services* created an organizing logic framework to illustrate how community-level factors influence health status. (See Figure 6.) They noted that disparities in access to health care; behaviors in response to illness; exposure to environmental and occupational hazards; health promotion and disease prevention behaviors; and experience of stress, societal support, and social cohesion all contribute to disparities in health status. Therefore, community-level interventions that address neighborhood conditions, employment opportunities, behavioral norms, opportunities for education and training, and access to health promotion, prevention, and care are key to addressing health disparities.[25] The model shows elements and associations at play in translating theory into research and action.

Diffusion of Innovations

In public health and health promotion, practitioners who want to make efficient use of resources must attend to the reach, adoption, implementation, and maintenance of programs. It is not enough to develop innovative programs; to reduce the burden of cancer, these programs must be disseminated widely. Cancer control measures will not realize their full potential for improving population health until effective programs are broadly diffused and disseminated. Multiple critiques, including one by the National Cancer Policy Board, suggest that failing to implement proven methods of cancer prevention and early detection results in tens of thousands of premature deaths each year.[26] Diffusion expands the number of people who are exposed to and reached by successful interventions, strengthening their public health impact.

Diffusion of Innovations Theory addresses how ideas, products, and social practices that are perceived as "new" spread throughout a society or from one society to another. According to the late E.M. Rogers, diffusion of innovations is "the process by which an *innovation* is communicated through certain *channels* over *time* among the members of a *social system*."[27] Diffusion Theory has been used to study the adoption of a wide range of health behaviors and programs, including condom use, smoking cessation, and use of new tests and technologies by health practitioners. Table 7. defines concepts that are central to this theory.

Diffusion of innovations that prevent disease and promote health requires a multilevel change process that usually takes place in

Table 7. Concepts in Diffusion of Innovations

Concept	Definition
Innovation	An idea, object, or practice that is thought to be new by an individual, organization, or community
Communication channels	The means of transmitting the new idea from one person to another
Social system	A group of individuals who together adopt the innovation
Time	How long it takes to adopt the innovation

diverse settings, through different strategies. At the individual level, adopting a health behavior innovation usually involves lifestyle change. At the organizational level, it may entail starting programs, changing regulations, or altering personnel roles. At a community level, diffusion can include using the media, advancing policies, or starting initiatives. According to Rogers, a number of factors determine how quickly, and to what extent, an innovation will be adopted and diffused. By considering the benefits of an innovation (see Table 8.), practitioners can position it effectively, thereby maximizing its appeal.

Specifically:

- *The relative advantage* of an innovation shows its superiority over whatever it replaces.

- *Compatibility* is an appropriate fit with the intended audience.

- *Complexity* has to do with how easy it is to implement the innovation.

- *Trialability* pertains to whether it can be tried on an experimental basis.

- *Observability* reflects whether the innovation will produce tangible results.

Effective diffusion requires practitioners to use both informal and formal communications channels and a spectrum of strategies for different settings. Disseminating an innovation in a variety of ways increases the likelihood that it will be adopted and *institutionalized*. Communication usually should include both mass media and interpersonal interactions. Through the *two-step flow of communication*, information from the media moves in two stages. First, opinion leaders, who pay close attention to the media, receive the information. Second, they convey their own interpretations, as well as the media content, to others. This process highlights the value of social networks for influencing adoption decisions.

Rogers described the process of adoption as a classic "bell curve," with five categories of adopters: *innovators*, *early adopters*, *early majority adopters*, *late majority adopters*, and *laggards*. When an innovation is introduced, the majority of people will either be early majority adopters or late majority adopters; fewer will be early adopters or laggards; and very few will be innovators (the first people to use the innovation). By identifying the

Table 8. Key Attributes Affecting the Speed and Extent of an Innovation's Diffusion

Attribute	Key Question
Relative advantage	Is the innovation better than what it will replace?
Compatibility	Does the innovation fit with the intended audience?
Complexity	Is the innovation easy to use?
Trialability	Can the innovation be tried before making a decision to adopt?
Observability	Are the results of the innovation observable and easily measurable?

> A university designs a program to help elementary school children cultivate healthy lifestyle habits and avoid chronic disease. The program has many components: it addresses the foods that children eat by modifying the fat and sugar content of school lunches, it teaches important health information through a classroom-based health education curriculum, and it encourages physical activity through a physical education component. It is highly successful; follow-up studies show that children who went through the program in elementary school continue to have healthier habits in their adolescence than those who did not go through the program.
>
> The fact that the program is successful is not enough to ensure it will change elementary school practices. To achieve a broader impact, the program must diffuse to other sites. Program planners may seek to demonstrate the *relative advantage* of the program by emphasizing its positive outcomes. They may try to show its *compatibility* by demonstrating that state policy-makers (e.g., the state Board of Education) have approved its materials. The program's *complexity* can be limited by creating user-friendly materials for teachers and cafeteria workers. By making the materials available on a Web site, they can enhance its *trialability*. Professional demonstrations of the program components can create an element of *observability*.

characteristics of people in each adopter category, practitioners can more effectively plan and implement strategies that are customized to their needs.

Communication Theory

Communication theory explores "who says what, in which channels, to whom, and with what effects." It investigates how messages are created, transmitted, received, and assimilated. When applied to public health problems, the central question theories of communication seek to answer is, "How do communication processes contribute to, or discourage, behavior change?" Focused on improving the health of communities rather than examining the underlying processes of communication, *public health communications* is the scientific development, strategic dissemination, and evaluation of relevant, accurate, accessible, and understandable health information, communicated to and from intended audiences to advance the public's health.[28]

Public health communications should represent an ecological perspective and foster multilevel strategies, such as tailored messages at the individual level, targeted messages at the group level, social marking at the community level, media advocacy at the policy level, and mass media campaigns at the population level.[29] Public health communications can increase knowledge and awareness of a health issue; influence perceptions, beliefs, and attitudes that factor into social norms; prompt action; demonstrate or illustrate healthy skills; increase support for services; debunk misconceptions; and strengthen organizational relations.[30] On the other hand, without supports in the social and physical environment, health communications alone may not be enough to sustain individual-level behavior changes, may not be effective for relaying complex health messages, and cannot compensate for lack of access to health care or healthy environments.[31]

Since other communication strategies are discussed elsewhere in this monograph, this section examines the role of mass media in public health interventions. The *media* are interconnected, large-scale organizations that gather, process, and disseminate news, information, entertainment, and advertising worldwide. Whether they are small operations, such as a neighborhood newspaper, or large corporations employing tens of thousands of people, the media influence almost every aspect of human life: economic, political, social, and behavioral.

Media Effects
The outcomes of media dissemination of ideas, images, themes, and stories are termed *media effects*. Media effects research investigates not only how the media influence the knowledge, opinions, attitudes, and behaviors of audience members, but also how audience members affect the media. Because audience members are active seekers and users of health information, the content transmitted through the media reflects their needs, interests, and preferences. Two questions are central to understanding the effects of media on audience members: 1) What factors affect the likelihood that a person will be exposed to a given message? 2) How do media effects vary with the amount of exposure to that message?[32]

Funding is a primary factor that determines whether or not audience members will be exposed to a message through the mass media, since money is needed to buy media time and space. Many public health programs do not have large budgets, so they often must rely on strategies for free distribution. Options may include public service announcements, embedding health messages in entertainment programs (e.g., soap operas), or promoting news coverage of public health topics in print and electronic media. Community institutions can adopt and disseminate messages, and social networks can also generate excitement about some messages, depending on their content.[33]

How often do people need to hear a message before it influences their beliefs or behaviors? This depends on several factors. Characteristics of target audiences (e.g., their readiness for change, the ways they process information), the complexity of the health issue, the presence of competing messages, and the nature of the health message influence the relationship between exposure to a health message and an outcome effect. Repeated exposure to a message, especially when it is delivered through multiple channels, may intensify its impact on audience members.[34]

Planners often assume that a certain percentage of the target audience will be exposed to a message and that another fraction of those who receive the message will be engaged by it. Yet there are several possible paths through which a health communications message can influence someone's beliefs and/or behaviors. These include *immediate learning* (people learn directly from the message), *delayed learning* (the impact of the message is not processed until some time after it has been conveyed), *generalized learning* (in addition to the message itself, people are persuaded about concepts related to the message), *social diffusion* (messages stimulate discussion among social groups, thereby affecting beliefs), and *institutional diffusion* (messages instigate a response from public institutions that reinforces the message's impact on the target audience.)[35]

Agenda Setting
The mass media can illuminate and focus attention on issues, helping to generate public awareness and momentum for change. A major focus of communications research

has been on how the mass media influence public opinion, especially about politics and policymaking. *Agenda setting* involves setting the media agenda (what is covered), the public agenda (what people think about), and the policy agenda (regulatory or legislative actions on issues).[36] (See Table 9.) Research on agenda setting has shown that the amount of media coverage an issue receives correlates strongly with the public's opinion of how important that issue is.

An axiom underlying this area of study is that mass media may not tell us *what* to think, but they are surprisingly effective in telling us what to think *about*. A critical construct of agenda setting, however, reinterprets this idea. *Framing* is a process in which someone tells the audience what aspect of the story is important. In other words, they tell the audience not only *what* to think about, but *how* to think about it. The way facts are packaged to tell a story creates the frame. By framing stories to emphasize social and environmental factors that affect health, public health advocates can use the media to pressure decision makers to develop and support healthy policies.

■ New Communication Technologies

New communication technologies have opened an extraordinary range of avenues for influencing health behavior. "E-health" (one element of new communication technologies) is the use of emerging information and communication technology, especially the Internet, to improve or enable

Table 9. Agenda Setting, Concepts, Definitions, and Applications

Concept	Definition	Potential Change Strategies
Media agenda setting	Institutional factors and processes influencing how the media define, select, and emphasize issues	Understand media professionals' needs and routines for gathering and reporting news
Public agenda setting	The link between issues covered in the media and the public's priorities	Use media advocacy or partnerships to raise public awareness of key health issues
Policy agenda setting	The link between issues covered in the media and the legislative priorities of policy makers	Advocate for media coverage to educate and pressure policy makers about changes to the physical and social environment needed to promote health
Problem definition	Factors and process leading to the identification of an issue as a "problem" by social institutions	Community leaders, advocacy groups, and organizations define an issue for the media and offer solutions
Framing	Selecting and emphasizing certain aspects of a story and excluding others	Advocacy groups "package" an important health issue for the media and the public

health and health care. The term refers to an emerging field in the intersection of medical informatics, public health, and business.[37] It bridges clinical and non-clinical sectors, and includes both individual and population health-oriented tools.[38] E-health communication strategies include, but are not limited to: health information on the Internet, online support groups, online collaborative communities, information tailored by computer technologies, educational computer games, computer-controlled in-home telephone counseling, and patient-provider e-mail contact.[39]

Major benefits of e-health strategies are increased reach (the ability to communicate to broad, geographically dispersed audiences), asynchronous communication (interaction not bounded by having to communicate at the same time) the ability to integrate multiple communication modes and formats (e.g., audio, video, text, graphics), the ability to track, preserve, and analyze communication (computer records of interaction, analysis of interaction trends), user control of the communication system (the ability to customize programs to user specifications), and interactivity (e.g., increased capacity for feedback).[40]

Educational and behavioral interventions employing new communication technologies are forging new ground and therefore benefit from the perspective provided by theories of health behavior. Like communications in other media, e-health interventions can address issues at the individual, group, or community/societal level; different theories may be appropriate, depending on the project's goals. For example, computer-tailored print materials encouraging individuals to eat more fruits and vegetables could be designed using the Stages of Change Model. Online support groups may apply theories of social support and social networks.

Community organizing approaches have been used to coordinate Internet-based campaigns through www.Meetup.com (a technology platform that helps people self-organize local gatherings).

Innovative e-health projects are expanding the range of tools that planners can use to develop cancer control and other interventions. For instance, NCI's Cancer Control Planet http://cancercontrolplanet.cancer.gov/ links public health professionals to comprehensive cancer control resources. NCI also has published data from its Health Information National Trends Survey (HINTS) on the Web at http://cancercontrol.cancer.gov/hints/. The HINTS program helps survey researchers, program planners, and social scientists understand how adults 18 years and older are using different communication channels, including the Internet. For example, according to recent HINTS data, when asked where they would go first if they had a strong need to get information about cancer, 34 percent of respondents said they would go to the Internet.

The HINTS data illustrate consumers' increasing reliance on the Internet as an easily accessible source of health information. The Internet has been characterized as a "hybrid technology" because it has the potential to reach millions of people with information that can be tailored to individual needs and preferences.[41] E-health interventions frequently offer information, education, and support directly to consumers. For example, the Association of Online Cancer Resources (ACOR), a collection of online communities designed to provide timely and accurate information in a supportive environment, is one case in point. ACOR delivers 1.8 million cancer messages each week (http://www.acor.org/).

Not all e-health interventions are Web-based. Computer applications have also allowed new uses of traditional health communications media, such as print and telephone. Tailored print communications (TPCs) and telephone-delivered interventions (TDIs) are two examples that have the potential for reaching linguistically and culturally diverse audiences. TPCs are printed materials created especially for an individual, based on relevant information about that person. Over 40 studies of TPCs have been conducted on a wide range of health topics, including diet, exercise, smoking cessation, mammography, and prostate cancer; most have found positive outcomes evidence. TDIs include a range of human-delivered counseling and reminder interventions delivered using the telephone and computer-generated voice response systems. Studies indicate that TDIs are effective across different populations and health topics, but do not have a broad-based reach. They have not been widely used by diverse populations.[42]

Interactive games offer another vehicle for intervention. Lieberman et al. designed a series of Nintendo video games to improve children's and adolescents' prevention and self care behaviors for asthma, diabetes, smoking prevention, and other health topics (see Figure 7.).[43] The games were based on well-established theories of learning and behavior change, such as Social Cognitive Theory. They reduced players' urgent care and emergency medical visits by as much as 77 percent.[44] Though research has demonstrated the effectiveness of some new communications technologies, further inquiry is needed into the mechanisms' underlying success.[45]

Opportunities are increasing for people to gain free access to the Internet via libraries and kiosks.[46] Unequal access remains problematic, however. Significant gaps in Internet usage between Caucasians, African Americans, and Hispanics persist,[47] and people with lower levels of educational attainment are also less likely to have Internet access. Because the Internet is a text-based medium, literacy issues that make it difficult for people to read print materials are also barriers to accessing Web-based information. There is danger that new computer technologies could worsen existing inequities in health status for diverse populations. It is therefore important to involve community members in planning e-health interventions and to offer them ongoing training and support for using these emerging communications tools.[48]

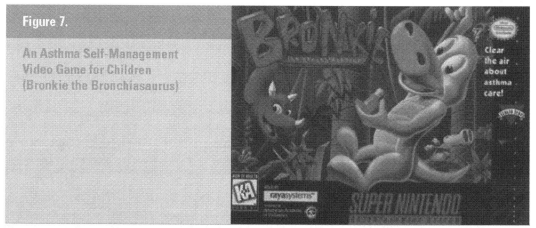

Figure 7.

An Asthma Self-Management Video Game for Children (Bronkie the Bronchiasaurus)

Box art reproduction used by permission of Health Hero Network. Copyright © 1994 by Health Hero Network. All rights reserved.

Part 3

Putting Theory And Practice Together

Planning Models

When practitioners begin the process of planning an intervention to promote health or change health behavior, theory helps them interpret the situation and guides their decisions about what design, procedures, and measurement indicators to select. Depending on the unit of practice (e.g., individuals, groups, organizations, community) and the nature of the health problem, different theoretical approaches may be appropriate. Practitioners can find that using more than one theory to address a problem produces a stronger impact. This is particularly true when planning comprehensive health promotion programs that address multiple levels (e.g., individual, organizational, community) of a health problem.

Planning models, such as PRECEDE-PROCEED and social marketing, help practitioners develop programs step by step, integrating multiple theories to explain and address health problems. Practitioners begin by using theory to develop a set of assumptions about factors contributing to a health problem. They then use research to test, adjust, and add to these assumptions. Armed with a theoretical framework and situation-specific research findings, practitioners design a targeted intervention strategy. This includes designing an evaluation to gauge whether or not the approach is effective, and choosing realistic, actionable goals that define in advance what programmatic success will look like.

Research (into the needs of the population, resources available, and the situation in which the health problem occurs) is a central feature of comprehensive planning models. Theory helps planners think about what questions to ask throughout program planning, implementation, and evaluation phases. During program planning, they explore the needs and resources of the population and learn how to design effective materials and strategies. During implementation, they seek to build and continually improve the program. After it ends, they assess what short-term and long-term effects the program has had on the health problem and its contributing factors.

Both social marketing and the PRECEDE-PROCEED model instruct the practitioner to begin the planning process by assessing the target audience's needs at multiple levels of a health problem. In social marketing, this preliminary investigation involves conducting consumer research and market analysis. In PRECEDE-PROCEED, it includes carrying out epidemiological assessment; behavioral, educational, environmental, and organizational diagnosis; and administrative and policy assessment. Both planning models combine behavior change theories for greater impact and use them as a basis for evaluation. These planning models are described in greater detail in the sections that follow.

Social Marketing

Social marketing uses marketing techniques to influence the voluntary behavior of target audience members for health benefit. It is distinct from health education in that it goes beyond informing or persuading people to reinforcing behavior with incentives and other benefits. It also differs from commercial marketing because the people who gain from it are members of the target audience. Another difference is that the marketing organization defines success in terms of positive effects on society.

Social marketing is not a theory, but an approach to promoting health behavior.

Alan Andreason defines it as "the application of commercial marketing technologies to the analysis, planning, execution, and evaluation of programs designed to influence the voluntary behavior of target audiences in order to improve their personal welfare and that of society."[49] This process creates a *voluntary exchange* between a marketing organization and members of a target audience based on mutual fulfillment of self-interest. In other words, the marketing organization exists to fulfill its mission (as defined by the organization's leadership), and the target audience members act in their own interests.

Social marketing programs are generally "consumer-driven," not expert-driven. They are targeted to serve a defined group of people. To avoid delineating the target market in an overly broad manner, social marketing practitioners *segment* a larger, heterogeneous target market into smaller subgroups. *Market segmentation* is the process of dividing a target audience into these more homogenous subgroups with distinct, unifying characteristics and needs. For example, factors such as regional location, ethnicity, gender, exercise habits, readiness for change, or media habits could be used to segment the larger audience of "smokers." Social marketing seeks to identify patterns that distinguish one target group from another to effectively target marketing strategies.

The social marketing process involves identifying an effective "marketing mix" ("The four Ps") of product, price, place, and promotion. The optimal marketing mix produces a timely exchange that heightens benefits, reduces barriers, and offers a better choice than the competition. The social marketer explores what benefits are of most interest to target market members and develops strategies and methods accordingly. The four Ps of the marketing mix are:

- *Product* (the right kind of behavioral change) includes not only the behavior that is being promoted, but also the benefits that go along with it.

- *Price* (an exchange of benefits and costs) refers to barriers or costs involved in adopting the behavior (e.g., money, time, effort).

- *Place* (making new behaviors easy to do) is about making the "product" accessible and convenient. It means delivering benefits in the right place at the right time.

- *Promotion* (delivering the message to the audience) is how the practitioner notifies the target market of the product, as well as its benefits, reasonable cost, and convenience.

Ideally, social marketing interventions begin with *formative research* (also called audience or consumer research) to understand the target market's perceptions, needs, and wants concerning the health behavior. Formative research includes learning about consumers' current behavior, what enables it, and what reinforces it. Practitioners also conduct a second type of research, *competitive analysis* (also called environmental analysis), to learn about the environment in which members of the target market are making behavior decisions. This analysis examines competing behaviors that are being promoted to the target market. (For example, messages encouraging people to eat convenient, inexpensive fast foods compete with messages about eating 5 fruits and vegetables a day.) It also investigates how consumers' decisions are shaped by factors such as their social and physical surroundings or their economic situation.

Evaluation is a critical and ongoing component of social marketing programs. Formative research helps practitioners to develop and refine concepts, messages, products, services, pricing, and distribution channels before they are fully implemented. Marketers often use qualitative methods, such as focus groups or key informant interviews, to pre-test marketing concepts, messages, and materials in a cost-effective manner. They may also pilot-test materials with individuals who share characteristics of the target market in order to verify their effectiveness, identify diverse channels for delivering the message, and measure outcomes. Process evaluation methods are used to track program outputs and processes during implementation. Social marketers also conduct summative research, often in the form of outcomes monitoring. This analysis compares the program's program objectives with its immediate and long-term outcomes to determine what worked, what didn't, and whether the program was cost-effective.

Social marketing programs are most successful when they are implemented using a research-driven process; then consumer research can help to adjust program messages and outputs. The social marketing process includes four stages: planning and strategy development; development of pretesting concepts, messages, and materials; implementation; assessment of in-market effectiveness; and feedback to the first stage. (See Figure 8.) Within each stage, there is a constant feedback loop between research and planning.

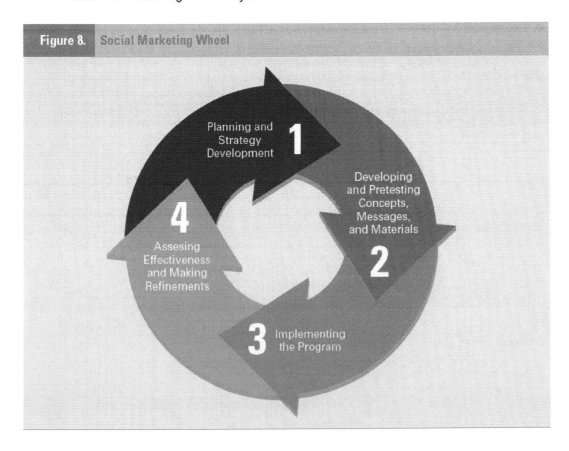

Figure 8. Social Marketing Wheel

1. Planning and Strategy Development
2. Developing and Pretesting Concepts, Messages, and Materials
3. Implementing the Program
4. Assesing Effectiveness and Making Refinements

As an approach that promotes behavior change through voluntary exchange and positive reinforcement, social marketing borrows substantively from behavior change theory. Behavioral theory offers insights into the current behavior of target market members and what might influence or change that behavior. For example, a social marketer who references Social Cognitive Theory might examine how self-efficacy and expectations about the outcome of a behavior factor into certain health practices within a target market.

The California 5 A Day Campaign, which was the model for the national 5 A Day program,[50] employs social marketing to increase Californians' consumption of fruit and vegetables through strategies such as supermarket point-of-purchase interventions, industry promotional support, media outreach, and community programs.[51] Several features of this program have been well-received.[52] First, it has a focused goal: to increase fruit and vegetable consumption by raising awareness of the health benefits. Second, its approach is built on an established theoretical framework—the Stages of Change model. Third, messages were designed and disseminated using consumer-driven communications strategies. Fourth, formative research (mall intercept interviews, focus groups, and baseline survey data) helped the planners to understand their audiences and improve messages. Lastly, the program uses the four Ps of social marketing:

- *Product:* Consuming more fruits and vegetables each day to minimize the risk of cancer and improve health status

- *Price:* The costs of eating a healthier diet (e.g., financial cost of buying fruits and vegetables, time cost of shopping for and preparing them, psychological cost of "worrying" about getting the recommended number of servings)

- *Place:* Grocery stores and other points of purchase (the 5 A Day message and healthy foods compete against unhealthy products for space and attention)

- *Promotion:* Branding the 5 A Day campaign to increase awareness (e.g., using a slogan and compelling images that are easy to recall)

Distribution channels include mass media advertising, public service announcements, newsletters, the Internet, magazines, press conferences, outreach activities, special events, and community-based groups, such as churches. Regular monitoring and evaluation help to assess the reach and impact of messages; efficient use of time, labor, and capital resources; and program costs/benefits.

PRECEDE-PROCEED

PRECEDE-PROCEED is a planning model, not a theory. It does not predict or explain factors linked to the outcomes of interest, but offers a framework for identifying intervention strategies to address these factors. Developed by Green, Kreuter, and associates,[53] PRECEDE-PROCEED provides a road map for designing health education and health promotion programs. It guides planners through a process that starts with desired outcomes and works backwards to identify a mix of strategies for achieving objectives. (See http://lgreen.net/index.html.)

Because the model views health behavior as influenced by both individual and environmental forces, it has two distinct parts: an "educational diagnosis"

(PRECEDE) and an "ecological diagnosis" (PROCEED). The PRECEDE acronym stands for Predisposing, Reinforcing, Enabling Constructs in Educational/Environmental Diagnosis and Evaluation. Developed in the 1970s, this component of the model posits that an educational diagnosis is needed to design a health promotion intervention, just as a medical diagnosis is needed to design a treatment plan. PROCEDE stands for Policy, Regulatory, and Organizational Constructs in Educational and Environmental Development. This element was added to the framework later, in 1991, to take into account the impact of environmental factors on health. Together, these two components of the model help practitioners plan programs that exemplify an ecological perspective.

PRECEDE-PROCEED has nine steps. The first five steps are diagnostic, addressing both educational and environmental issues. These include: (1) social assessment, (2) epidemiological assessment, (3) behavioral and environmental assessment, (4) educational and ecological assessment, and (5) administrative and policy assessment. The last four comprise implementation and evaluation of health promotion intervention. These include: (6) implementation, (7) process evaluation, (8) impact evaluation, and (9) outcome evaluation. (See Figure 9.)

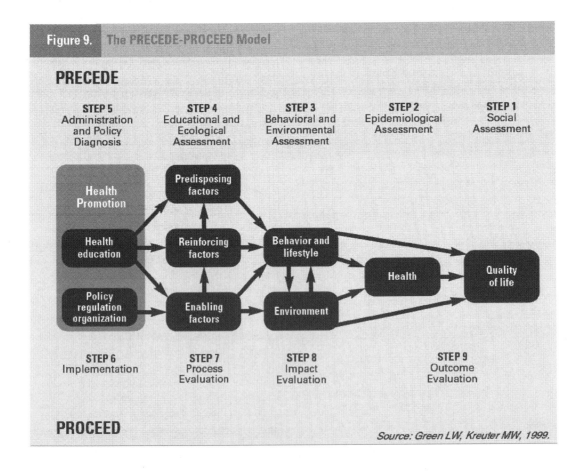

Figure 9. The PRECEDE-PROCEED Model

Source: Green LW, Kreuter MW, 1999.

During the diagnostic steps of the model, practitioners employ various methods to learn about the community's perceived and actual needs, as well as the regulatory context in which the intervention will operate. To conduct *social assessment*, the practitioner may use multiple data collection activities (e.g., key informant interviews, focus groups, participant observation, surveys) to understand the community's perceived needs. *Epidemiological assessment* may include secondary data analysis or original data collection to prioritize the community's health needs and establish program goals and objectives. *Behavioral and Environmental Assessment* identifies factors, both internal and external to the individual, that affect the health problem. Reviewing the literature and applying theory are two ways to map out these factors.

In *Educational and Ecological Assessment*, the practitioner identifies antecedent and reinforcing factors that must be in place to initiate and sustain change. Behavior—such as reducing intake of dietary fat, engaging in routine physical activity, and obtaining annual mammograms—is shaped by predisposing, reinforcing, and enabling factors. Practitioners can use individual, interpersonal, or community-level change theories to classify determinants of behavior into one of these three categories and rank their importance. Because each type of factor requires different intervention strategies, classifying them helps practitioners consider how to address community needs. The three types of influencing factors include:

- *Predisposing factors*, which motivate or provide a reason for behavior; they include knowledge, attitudes, cultural beliefs, and readiness to change.

- *Enabling factors*, which enable persons to act on their predispositions; these factors include available resources, supportive policies, assistance, and services.

- *Reinforcing factors*, which come into play after a behavior has been initiated; they encourage repetition or persistence of behaviors by providing continuing rewards or incentives. Social support, praise, reassurance, and symptom relief might all be considered reinforcing factors.

In the final diagnostic step of PRECEDE-PROCEED, *Administrative and Policy Assessment*, intervention strategies reflect information gathered in previous steps; the availability of needed resources; and organizational policies and regulations that could affect program implementation. (See Table 10.)

The four remaining steps of PRECEDE-PROCEED comprise program implementation and evaluation. Before *Implementation* (Step 6) begins, practitioners should prepare plans for evaluating the process (Step 7), impact (Step 8), and outcome (Step 9) of the intervention. *Process Evaluation* gauges the extent to which a program is being carried out according to plan. *Impact Evaluation* looks at changes in factors (i.e., predisposing, enabling, and reinforcing factors) that influence the likelihood that behavioral and environmental change will occur. Lastly, *outcome evaluation* looks at whether the intervention has affected health and quality-of-life indicators.

As Table 11 shows, the individual, interpersonal, and community-level theories discussed in this monograph are most useful when applied to PRECEDE-PROCEED's diagnostic steps. Community organization relates to Step 1, which may entail working with communities to identify their own needs, strengths, resources, and capacities. Descriptive epidemiology is most pertinent to Step 2, but community-level theories may be relevant if the community helps to choose the health problem that will be addressed, or to set priorities among health problems. Theory is most directly useful when applied to steps 3, 4, and 5, since these steps call upon the practitioner to make strategic decisions. By using theory, the practitioner can make sound choices that are based upon more than just intuition and personal judgment.

Theory should guide practitioners' examination of predisposing, enabling, and reinforcing factors. For example, the Health Belief Model suggests that certain beliefs might influence women's decisions about whether or not to get a mammogram, such as perceived chances of developing cancer (perceived susceptibility), or how serious they believe cancer would be (perceived severity). Both beliefs constitute predisposing factors. Other HBM constructs may identify possible perceived benefits of and barriers to screening. Receiving

Table 10. Diagnostic Elements of PRECEDE-PROCEED

Planning Step	Function	Examples of Relevant Theory
1. Social Assessment	Assesses people's views of their own needs and quality of life	Community organization Community building
2. Epidemiological Assessment	Documents which health problems are most important for which groups in a community	Community-level theories (If the community helps to choose the health problem that will be addressed)
3. Behavioral/ Environmental Assessment	Identifies factors that contribute to the health problem of interest	Interpersonal theories - Social Cognitive Theory Theories of organizational change Community organization Diffusion of innovations
4. Educational/ Ecological Assessment	Identifies preceding and reinforcing factors that must be in place to initiate and sustain change	All three levels of change theories: - Individual - Interpersonal - Community
5. Administrative/ Policy Assessment	Identifies policies, resources, and circumstances in the program's context that may help or hinder implementation	Community-level theories: - Community organization - Organizational change

reassurance that they do not have cancer (perceived benefit) might be a reinforcing factor. Lack of insurance coverage for screening mammography (perceived barrier) could be a negative enabling factor.

By exploring the degree to which each of these factors affects women's behaviors, program planners can decide how to focus program messages for a communications campaign or strategies for an administrative intervention (such as providing low- or no-cost screening or changing insurance coverage). The best way to verify and rank explanations offered by theory is to gather information directly from women in the target population. Another, less ideal approach is to learn by reading research literature on women who share characteristics with the target population.

Where to Begin: Choosing the Right Theories

Interventions that evolve from a comprehensive planning process, build on prior research, and use health behavior theories are more likely to be effective. By investigating what factors influence the target population's behavior, including their social and physical environments, practitioners gain the raw materials they need to meet the needs of that population. Theory helps practitioners to interpret the findings of their research, making the leap from facts on a page to understanding the dynamic interactions between behavior and environmental context. Systematic approaches to tailoring, targeting, implementing, and evaluating programs provide practitioners with a framework for translating this insight into actions that improve health outcomes.

To make appropriate use of theory in a given situation, practitioners must consider both the social or health problem at hand and the context in which the intervention will take place. Once they have identified a problem, they can use a planning system such as social marketing or PRECEDE-PROCEED to identify social science theories that contribute to their understanding. These theories can guide them to potential points of intervention. Consulting the research literature helps practitioners to learn about the past successes or failures of intervention strategies that they consider, and reflect on whether those strategies are likely to work for the current situation. Pre-testing and actively discussing proposed strategies with the target audience can also help to determine whether or not they will be well received.

Table 11. summarizes the focus and key concepts of each of the eight theories described in this guide. Refer to this table to identify theories that help explain and address a health problem. For example, several theories could be used to inform the design of a program to reduce tobacco use among adolescents. By scanning the "Focus" column, one can quickly gauge which theories might apply to a particular situation. For example, The Stages of Change model might be very useful, since it centers on individuals' readiness to change. On the other hand, the Health Belief Model seems less promising, since young people may be less concerned about long-term health problems. (In fact, they may not feel vulnerable to disease at all!) Social Cognitive Theory could be helpful because it emphasizes the interplay between personal, environmental, and behavior factors. Likewise, Community Organization could offer perspective on activating young people around tobacco control issues. Applying each of these theories might look like this:

- *Stages of Change:* Learn more about readiness to change among adolescents who smoke in order to plan appropriate and effective cessation messages and strategies.

- *Social Cognitive Theory:* Examine how social environment, including peer attitudes, influences adolescents' tobacco use. What are the expectations of teens who experiment with tobacco, or who use it regularly? How do observational learning and reinforcement contribute to the reasons why they smoke? Might these constructs help identify someone who can successfully help them to quit?

- *Community Organization:* Consider how to involve teen smokers in developing and carrying out the program. One idea might be to organize a coalition of concerned parents, teachers, and teens to help explore why teens smoke, and identify potential solutions.

The examples above offer a basic illustration of how multiple theories might be combined to address a single problem. The resulting program would be a multi-faceted, multilevel effort.

■ A Few Final Words

Once one is familiar with some contemporary theories of health behavior, the challenge is to use them appropriately within a comprehensive planning process. Planning systems, such as social marketing and PRECEDE-PROCEED, facilitate the process of developing successful programs because they lead practitioners through a step-by-step process of examining health and behavior at multiple levels.

At the most basic level, an ecological perspective points to two approaches to addressing health problems: change people's behavior or change the environment. The most powerful health promotion and behavior change interventions integrate these approaches and treat them both as essential. Figure 10. illustrates that strategies intended to change *people's behavior* can often be derived from individual-level theories; those aimed at changing the *environment* draw on community-level theories. Theories at the interpersonal level (such as Social Cognitive Theory) lie in-between, exploring the reciprocal exchanges between individuals and their environments.

Practitioners who are aware of reciprocal causation (i.e., that individual behavior both influences, and is influenced by, the environment) are more likely to design multidimensional, effective health promotion programs. A change strategy based on individual-level theory may indirectly lead to changes in the environment (e.g., when individuals' improved eating habits drive the cafeteria to offer healthier choices). By the same token, a strategy based on community-level theory may yield improved individual health behaviors (e.g., when an individual's involvement in a community organizing project to improve access to fruits and vegetables in the community inspires her to cook healthier foods for her family).

Theoretical frameworks offer flexible guidance for applying the abstract concepts of theory to a vast array of real circumstances. By becoming familiar with

Table 11. Summary of Theories: Focus and Key Concepts

	Theory	Focus	Key Concepts
Individual Level	Health Belief Model	Individuals' perceptions of the threat posed by a health problem, the benefits of avoiding the threat, and factors influencing the decision to act	Perceived susceptibility Perceived severity Perceived benefits Perceived barriers Cues to action Self-efficacy
	Stages of Change Model	Individuals' motivation and readiness to change a problem behavior	Precontemplation Contemplation Decision Action Maintenance
	Theory of Planned Behavior	Individuals' attitudes toward a behavior, perceptions of norms, and beliefs about the ease or difficulty of changing	Behavioral intention Attitude Subjective norm Perceived behavioral control
	Precaution Adoption Process Model	Individuals' journey from lack of awareness to action and maintenance	Unaware of issue Unengaged by issue Deciding about acting Deciding not to act Deciding to act Acting Maintenance
Interpersonal Level	Social Cognitive Theory	Personal factors, environmental factors, and human behavior exert influence on each other	Reciprocal determinism Behavioral capability Expectations Self-efficacy Observational learning Reinforcements
Community Level	Community Organization	Community-driven approaches to assessing and solving health and social problems	Empowerment Community capacity Participation Relevance Issue selection Critical consciousness
	Diffusion of Innovations	How new ideas, products, and practices spread within a society or from one society to another	Relative advantage Compatibility Complexity Trialability Observability
	Communication Theory	How different types of communication affect health behavior	Example: *Agenda Setting* Media agenda setting Public agenda setting Policy agenda setting Problem identification, definition Framing

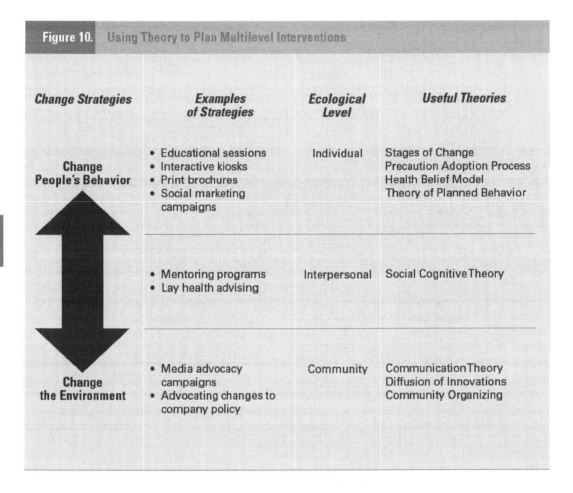

Figure 10. Using Theory to Plan Multilevel Interventions

Change Strategies	Examples of Strategies	Ecological Level	Useful Theories
Change People's Behavior	• Educational sessions • Interactive kiosks • Print brochures • Social marketing campaigns	Individual	Stages of Change Precaution Adoption Process Health Belief Model Theory of Planned Behavior
	• Mentoring programs • Lay health advising	Interpersonal	Social Cognitive Theory
Change the Environment	• Media advocacy campaigns • Advocating changes to company policy	Community	Communication Theory Diffusion of Innovations Community Organizing

behavior change theories and planning systems, practitioners gain access to tools that allow them to generate creative solutions to unique situations. They are able to go beyond acting on instinct or repeating earlier interventions to adopt a systematic, scientific approach to their work. Theory helps practitioners to ask the right questions and effective planning helps them zero in on factors that contribute to a problem. Other key elements of effective programs include matching programs to the audience, making information accessible and practical, involving participants in active learning, and including elements that build skills and reinforce behavior change.

Becoming comfortable with behavior change theory as an instrument of practice may take some work, but the results are well worth it. Behavior change theory is not simply a tool for academics and researchers; it can be applied to the problems health promotion practitioners face every day. The abstractions of theory help practitioners to understand the dynamics underlying real situations and to think about solutions in a new way. Armed with this resource, you may find yourself saying, as did Winston Churchill in 1898, "I pass with relief from the tossing sea of Cause and Theory to the firm ground of Result and Fact."

PART 3

47

PUTTING THEORY AND PRACTICE TOGETHER

Sources

Bandura A. Social Foundations of Thought and Action: A Social Cognitive Theory. Englewood Cliffs, N.J.: Prentice-Hall, 1986.

Glanz K, Rimer BK, Lewis FM. Health Behavior and Health Education: Theory, Research, and Practice (3rd Edition). San Francisco, Calif.: Jossey-Bass, 2002.

Prochaska JO, DiClemente CC, Norcross JC. In Search of How People Change: Applications to the Addictive Behaviors. American Psychologist 47:1102–1114, 1992.

Rosenstock IM, Strecher VJ, Becker MH. Social Learning Theory and the Health Belief Model. Health Education Quarterly 15(2):175–183, 1988.

van Ryn M, Heaney CA. Developing Effective Helping Relationships in Health Education Practice. Health Education and Behavior 24:683–702, 1997.

Kotler P, Andreasen A. Strategic Marketing for Nonprofit Organizations (5th Edition). Prentice-Hall, 1996.

Office of Cancer Communications, National Cancer Institute. Making Health Communication Programs Work: A Planner's Guide (revised December 2001). NIH Pub. No. 02-5145, 2002.

Glanz, Karen and Rimer, Barbara K. *Theory at a Glance*: A Guide for Health Promotion Practice. National Cancer Institute, National Institutes of Health, U.S. Department of Health and Human Services. NIH Pub. No. 97-3896. Washington, DC: NIH, Revised September 1997.

References

[1] Glanz K, Rimer BK, Lewis FM. Health Behavior and Health Education: Theory, Research, and Practice (3rd Edition). San Francisco, Calif.: Jossey-Bass, 2002.

[2] Institute of Medicine. Speaking of Health: Assessing Health Communications Strategies for Diverse Populations. Washington, D.C.: National Academies Press, 2002.

[3] Kreuter MW, Skinner CS. Tailoring: what's in a name? Health Education Research 15(1):1, 2000.

[4] McLeroy KR, Bibeau D, Steckler A, Glanz K. An ecological perspective on health promotion programs. Health Education Quarterly 15:351–377, 1988.

[5] Office on Smoking and Health, National Center for Chronic Disease Prevention and Health Promotion, Centers for Disease Control and Prevention, U.S. Department of Health and Human Services. Best Practices for Comprehensive Tobacco Control Programs. Atlanta Ga.: August 1999.

[6] Prochaska JO, DiClemente CC. Stages and processes of self-change of smoking: Toward an integrative model of change. Journal of Consulting and Clinical Psychology 51(3): 390–395, 1983.

[7] Azjen I, Driver BL. Prediction of leisure participation from behavioral, normative, and control beliefs: an application of the theory of planned behavior. Leisure Science 13:185–204, 1991.

[8] Mandelblatt JS, Gold K, O'Malley AS, et al. Breast and cervix cancer screening among multiethnic women: Role of age, health, and source of care. Preventive Medicine 28:418–425, 1999.

[9] Institute of Medicine, op. cit.

[10] Baranowski T, et al. Increasing fruit and vegetable consumption among 4th and 5th grade students: results from focus groups using reciprocal determinism. Journal of Nutrition Education 25:114–327, 1993.

[11] Lorig K, Sobel D, Stewart A, et al. Evidence suggesting that a chronic disease self-management program can improve health status while reducing hospitalization. Medical Care 37(1):5–14, 1999.

[12] Fetterman DM, Kaftarian SJ, Wandersman A. Empowerment Evaluation: Knowledge and Tools for Self-assessment and Accountability. Thousand Oaks, Calif.: Sage Publications, 1996.

[13] Fawcett SB, Francisco VT, Schultz JA, et al. The Community Tool Box: A Web-Based Resource for Building Healthier Communities. Public Health Rep. 115(2-3):274–8, Mar-Jun, 2000.

[14] Rothman J. Approaches to Community Intervention. In Rothman J, Erlich JL, Tropman JE (eds.), Strategies of Community Intervention. Itasca, Ill.: Peacock Publishers, 2001.

[15] Wallerstein N. Powerlessness, empowerment, and health: implications for health promotion programs. American Journal of Health Promotion 6:197–205, 1992.

[16] Fisher R. Social Action Community Organization: Proliferation, Persistence, Roots, and Prospects. In Minkler M (ed.), Community Organizing and Community Building for Health. Rutgers, N.J.: Rutgers University Press, 1997.

[17] Alinsky SD. Rules for Radicals. New York, N.Y.: Vintage Books, 1989.

[18] Parachini L, Covington S. Community Organizing Toolbox: A Funder's Guide to Community Organizing Neighborhood Funders Group. Washington, D.C.: April 2001.
URL: http://www.aecf.org/tarc/publications/pubs_toolbox.php

[19] Alinsky, op. cit.

[20] Dorfman L, Wallack L, Themba M. Media Advocacy and Public Health: Power for Prevention. Newbury Park, Calif.: Sage Publications, 1993.

[21] Wallack L., Dorfman L. Issue 1. Berkeley Media Studies Group, Berkeley, CA. January, 1997.

[22] Nichter M. Project community diagnosis: Participatory research as a first step toward community involvement in primary health care in Hahn RA (ed.), Anthropology in public health: Bridging the differences in culture and society. New York, N.Y.: Oxford University Press, 1999.

[23] Thompson B, Nettekoven L, Ferster D, Stanley LC, Thompson J, Corbett KK. Chapter 5: Mobilizing the COMMIT Communities for Smoking Control. Smoking and Tobacco Control Monograph 6: Community-Based Interventions for Smokers: The COMMIT Field Experience. Tobacco Control Research Branch, Division of Cancer Control and Population Sciences, National Cancer Institute, National Institutes of Health. 1993.

[24] Community-based interventions for smokers: The COMMIT Field Experience, Smoking and Tobacco Control Monograph No. 6. Burns D, Garfinkel L, Samet J, editors. USDHHS NIH NCI. NIH Publication No. 95-4028, 1995.

[25] Institute of Medicine, op. cit.

[26] National Cancer Policy Board, Institute of Medicine. Fulfilling the Potential of Cancer Prevention and Early Detection. Washington, D.C.: The National Academies Press, 2003.

[27] Rogers EM. Diffusion of Innovations (4th Edition). New York, N.Y.: Free Press, 1995.

[28] Bernhardt JM. Communication at the Core of Public Health. American Journal of Public Health 94(12): 2051–2052, December 2004.

[29] Ibid.

[30] Office of Cancer Communications, National Cancer Institute. Making Health Communication Programs Work: A Planner's Guide (revised December 2001). NIH Pub. No. 02-5145, 2002.

[31] Freimuth V, Quinn SC. The Contributions of Health Communication to Eliminating Health Disparities. American Journal of Public Health 94(12):2053–2054, December 2004.

[32] Institute of Medicine, op. cit.

[33] Freimuth V, Quinn SC, op. cit.

[34] Ibid.

[35] Ibid.

[36] Dorfman L, Wallack L, Themba M, op cit.

[37] Eysenbach G. What is e-health? Journal of Medical Internet Research 3(2):e20, 2001. URL: http://www.jmir.org/20012/e20

[38] Eng TR. The eHealth Landscape: A Terrain Map of Emerging Information and Communication Technologies in Health and Health Care. The Robert Woods Johnson Foundation, 2001. URL: http://www.informatics-review.com/thoughts/rwjf.html

[39] Neuhauser L, Kreps G. Rethinking Communication in the E-health Era. Journal of Health Psychology 8(1): 7–22, 2003.

[40] Science Panel on Interactive Communication and Health. Wired for Health and Well-Being: The Emergence of Interactive Health Communications. U.S. Department of Health and Human Services, U.S. Government Printing Office. Washington, D.C.: April 1999. URL: http://www.health.gov/scipich/pubs/finalreport.htm

[41] Cassell MM, Jackson C, Cheuvront B. Health communication on the Internet: an effective channel for health behavior change? J Health Commun 3(1):71-9, Jan-Mar 1998.

[42] Institute of Medicine, op. cit.

[43] Lieberman, D.A. Interactive video games for health promotion: Effects on knowledge, self-efficacy, social support, and health. R.L. Street, W.R. Gold, & T. Manning (Eds.), Health promotion and interactive technology: Theoretical applications and future directions. Mahwah, NJ: Lawrence Erlbaum Associates, pp. 103–120, 1997.

[44] Lieberman DA. Management of chronic pediatric diseases with interactive health games: Theory and research findings. Journal of Ambulatory Care Management 24(1):26–38, 2001.

[45] Kreps GL. Evaluating new health information technologies: expanding the frontiers of health care delivery and health promotion. Stud Health Technol Inform 80:205–12, 2002.

[46] U.S. Department of Commerce. A Nation On-line: How Americans are Expanding their Use of the Internet. Economics and Statistics Administration, National Telecommunications and Information Administration. February 2002. URL: http://www.ntia.doc.gov/ntiahome/dn/anationonline2.pdf

[47] Leslie Harris & Associates. Bringing a Nation On-line: The Importance of Federal Leadership. The Leadership Conference on Civil Rights Education Fund and the Benton Foundation. July 2002. URL: http://www.benton.org/publibrary/nationonline/bringing_a_nation.pdf

[48] Institute of Medicine, op cit.

[49] Andreasen A. Marketing Social Change: Changing Behavior to Promote Health, Social Development, and the Environment. San Francisco, Calif.: Jossey-Bass, 1995.

[50] National Cancer Institute. 5 A Day for Better Health Program, Chapter 1. National Institutes of Health. NIH Pub. No. 01-5019. Washington, DC: September 2001.

[51] California Department of Health Services. Cancer Prevention and Nutrition Section. Eat 5 A Day for Better Health. 2005. URL: http://www.dhs.ca.gov/ps/cdic/cpns/ca5aday/

[52] Alcalay R, Bell R. Promoting Nutrition and Physical Activity Through Social Marketing. Department of Communication and the Center for Advanced Studies in Nutrition and Social Marketing. University of California, Davis, June, 2000.
http://socialmarketing-nutrition.ucdavis.edu/publications.htm

[53] Green LW, Kreuter MW. Health Promotion Planning: An Educational and Ecological Approach (3rd edition). McGraw-Hill, 1999.

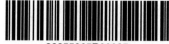

Made in the USA
San Bernardino, CA
24 January 2019